Imen Sellami
Anwar Abbes
Afef Feki

Workload and smoking in the workplace

Imen Sellami
Anwar Abbes
Afef Feki

Workload and smoking in the workplace

A factor that encourages smoking

ScienciaScripts

Imprint

Any brand names and product names mentioned in this book are subject to trademark, brand or patent protection and are trademarks or registered trademarks of their respective holders. The use of brand names, product names, common names, trade names, product descriptions etc. even without a particular marking in this work is in no way to be construed to mean that such names may be regarded as unrestricted in respect of trademark and brand protection legislation and could thus be used by anyone.

Cover image: www.ingimage.com

This book is a translation from the original published under ISBN 978-620-6-71337-1.

Publisher:
Sciencia Scripts
is a trademark of
Dodo Books Indian Ocean Ltd. and OmniScriptum S.R.L publishing group

120 High Road, East Finchley, London, N2 9ED, United Kingdom
Str. Armeneasca 28/1, office 1, Chisinau MD-2012, Republic of Moldova, Europe
Printed at: see last page
ISBN: 978-620-7-66323-1

THE BURDEN OF AND SMOKING IN THE WORKPLACE

A FACTOR THAT ENCOURAGES SMOKING

TABLE OF CONTENTS

INTRODUCTION

Tobacco use remains a major public health concern, representing a persistent challenge worldwide. Despite numerous awareness, prevention and cessation initiatives, tobacco use remains a prevalent public health problem affecting millions of people worldwide [1].

The persistence of smoking on a global scale is a cause for concern because of the multiple harmful consequences it has on individual and collective health. Tobacco-related diseases, such as cardiovascular disease, cancer, respiratory disease and other health disorders, impose a considerable burden on national health systems. The medical costs associated with treating these diseases, as well as lost productivity due to work absenteeism and disability, have a significant economic impact worldwide [1].

It is one of the leading risk factors for death worldwide, mainly ischaemic heart disease and cancer [2,3].

Tunisia has not been spared from this scourge [4]. Tobacco control is one of the priorities of public health programmes, which focus on informing the general population about the risks of smoking [5].

In the workplace, smoking can damage the health not only of smokers but also of those around them. In addition, certain working conditions and physical or psychosocial risk factors seem to be associated with an increase in smoking, which is why companies, through the occupational health physician, are implementing strategies to reduce smoking in the workplace. prevention of health risk behaviours, the most worrying of which remains the fight against smoking in the workplace [6].

In this approach, the occupational physician is a key player in the development of the tobacco control strategy. They are in the best position to assess the prevalence of smoking in the workplace and to understand the relationship between workers' nicotine dependence and perceived workload, and consequently to develop appropriate and effective interventions [7,8].

In this context, we set ourselves the objectives of assessing the prevalence of smoking in an electricity and gas company in the Sfax region and of studying the relationship between workers' nicotine dependence and the perceived workload likely to guide anti-smoking measures.

METHODS

1. NATURE OF THE STUDY

We conducted a descriptive and analytical cross-sectional study from July to December 2022.

2. POPULATION OF THE STUDY

The study concerned electrical technicians from an electricity and gas company who agreed to take part in our survey.

Incomplete forms were excluded from the survey.

3. METHODS

3.1. Collection of data

The study can only be carried out with the authorisation of the company's medical department management, which is convinced of the study's objectives and its impact on staff activity. We worked with the company's occupational physicians to distribute the self-completed questionnaire during the periodic check-ups of electrical technicians.

3.2. The questionnaire

Data were collected using a questionnaire consisting of two parts parties. The first part was completed by the participants. This part assessed employees' socio-demographic and occupational data, as well as their smoking habits.The second part was completed by the interviewer concerning the perceived workload. of work.

4. THE VARIABLES STUDIED

* Smoking behaviour :

Smoking behaviour included smoking habits, the variety and quantity of tobacco consumed and smoking dependence assessed by the Arabic version of the Fagerström test (0-2 points: no nicotine dependence, 3-4 points: low nicotine dependence, 5-6 points: moderate nicotine dependence, 7-8 points: high nicotine dependence and 9-10 points: very high nicotine dependence) [9].

* Perceived workload :

Perceived workload was assessed using the Raw National Aeronautics and Space Administration Task Load Index (raw NASA-TLX) questionnaire. This scale is made up of six criteria, namely the requirement to physical demands, time demands, effort, the need to be on the ball performance and frustration. For each of the six questions corresponding to these criteria, the participants were asked to answer with a score from 0, indicating a low level, to 100, indicating a high level of this criterion. The workload was obtained by calculating the average of the scores for each of the six criteria [10,11]. The overall raw TLX score is an average of the scores for each of the six criteria.

5. ETHICAL CONSIDERATIONS

The free participation of staff in our study was a principle, reflecting our commitment to research ethics. The decision to contribute to our survey was entirely voluntary, and no participant was put under any pressure. This approach aimed to ensure that individuals made a genuine commitment, which contributes to the reliability and validity of the data collected.The process of collecting and interpreting the data was carried out in strict confidentiality. All the information gathered was treated anonymously, excluding any possibility of individual identification. This confidentiality measure was put in place to preserve the integrity and privacy of the participants, thereby reinforcing confidence in the research process. In addition, we would like to emphasise that our research team officially declares the absence of any conflict of interest in this study. This Transparency is essential to establish the credibility of our results and demonstrate the objectivity of our scientific approach. Our research did not involve any financial, professional or personal links likely to influence the results in a biased way.

6. ANALYSIS STATISTICS

The data was entered into an Excel 2010 spreadsheet. Data analysis was carried out using the $20^{\text{ème}}$ version of SPSS (Statistical Package for the Social Sciences). We divided our population into 2 groups: a non-smoking group comprising participants who had never smoked and ex-smokers, and a group comprising current smokers.

6.1. Descriptive study :

We calculated frequencies and percentages for the qualitative variables.Means and standard deviations were used to describe the quantitative variables.

6.2. Analytical study

For the bivariate analytical study, we used Pearson's correlation coefficient to study the relationship between the Fagerström score and the score of each criterion of the NASA-TLX raw. For all statistical tests, the p significance level was set at 0.05.

RESULTS

Eighty-two male employees took part in our study.

1. SOCIO-DEMOGRAPHIC DATA :

1.1. Breakdown by marital status :

Of our participants, 57 electrical technicians (69.5%) were married (Figure 1).

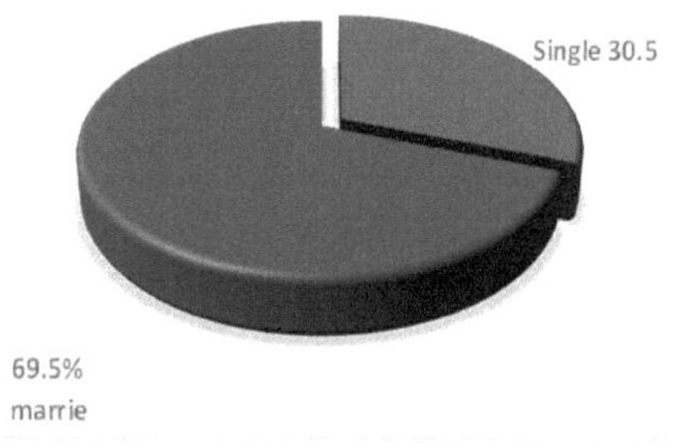

Figure 1: Breakdown of participants by marital status

1.2. Breakdown by age

The mean age was 38.4 ± 10.12 years.

1.3. Breakdown by level of education

Of our participants, 84.2% had secondary education (Figure 2).

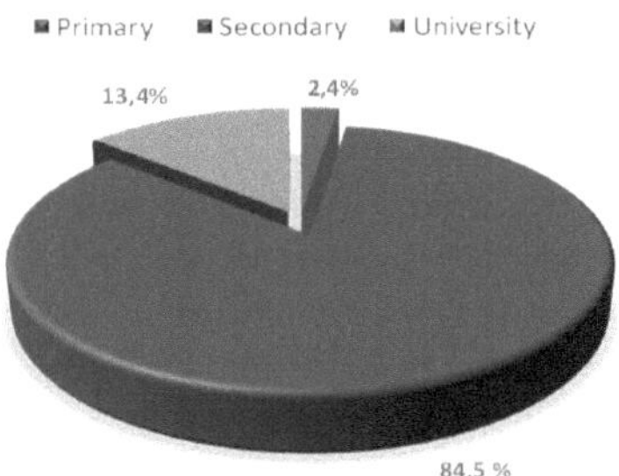

Figure 2: Breakdown of participants by level of education

1.4. Habits of life

The prevalence of smoking among participants was 45.1% (Figure 3).

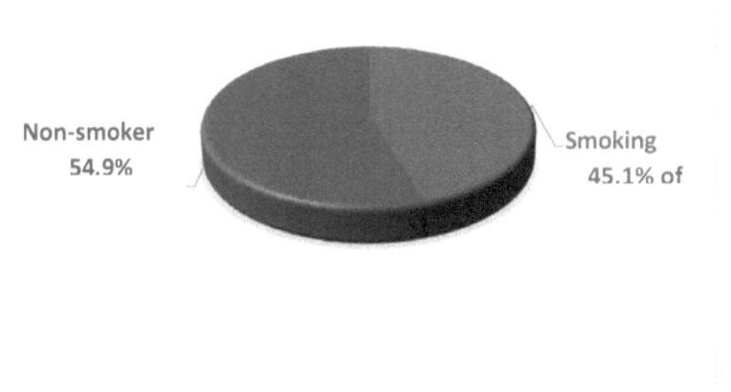

Figure 3: Breakdown of participants by smoking status

Consumption in pack-years was 13.28±10.72. We found that 7 participants used chicha, i.e. 8.5% of the study population. The average consumption of chicha was 3 ± 3 chichas per week. No participants reported using Neffa or illicit products.

1.5. Sports activity

Sport was practised by 47.5% of participants, compared with 52.5% who did not practise sport.

1.6. Body mass index

The average body mass index was $27.1\pm5.6 \ kg/m^2$.

2. DATA PROFESSIONAL

2.1. Breakdown by professional category

Of our participants, 22% were senior technicians (Table I).

Table I: Distribution of participants by professional category

(n=82)

Professional categories	Number	Percentage (%)
Technical assistant	13	15 ,9
Team Leader	11	13,4
Against master	6	7,3
Head of department	3	3,7
Qualified line fitter	23	28
Skilled worker	3	3,7
Lifter	1	1,2
Cutter	2	2,4
Senior technician	2	2,4
Senior technician	18	22
Total	82	100

2.2. Length of service

The average length of service was 14.7±11.2 years.

2.3. Breakdown by perceived workload at work

We found that the overall raw TLX score was 69.2±24.9 (Table II).

Table II: Perceived workload (n=82)

NASA-TLX* raw criteria	Mean ± Standard deviation
Mental demands	88,8±13,5
Physical requirements	63,6±24,7
Time requirement	59,1±28,4
Effort	83,8±14
Performance	85,4±13,1
Frustration	34,5±28,1
Overall score for raw TLX	69,2±24,9

3. DEPENDENCE A THE NICOTINE AT THE SMOKING PARTICIPANTS

3.1. Distribution of responses to thetest in participants who smoke

Among our participants, 48.7% smoked within 30 minutes of waking up, while 40.5% took cigarettes at shorter intervals during the first hours of the morning (Table III).

Table III: Distribution of responses to the Fagerström test in participants who smoke (n=37)

Variables							Number	Percentage (%)
Time to smoke after waking up								
Within 5 minutes							3	8,2
6-30 minutes							15	40,5
31-60 minutes							5	13,5
More than 60 minutes							14	37,8
The difficulty of smoking in places where prohibited								
Yes							9	24,4
No							28	75,6
Cigarettes are hard to quit								
First of the day							19	51,3
To another							18	48,7
Number of cigarettes per day								
10 or less							14	37,8
11 à 20							18	48,6
21 à 30							5	13,6
Smoking at shorter intervals in the early hours of the morning								
Yes							15	40,5
No							22	59,5
Smoking when you are so ill								
to have	stay	at	bed	almost	any	the		
day								
Yes							13	35,1
No							24	64,9

3.2. Nicotine dependence at participants

Nicotine dependence assessed by the Fagerström test was moderate to high in 40.5% of smokers (Figure 4).

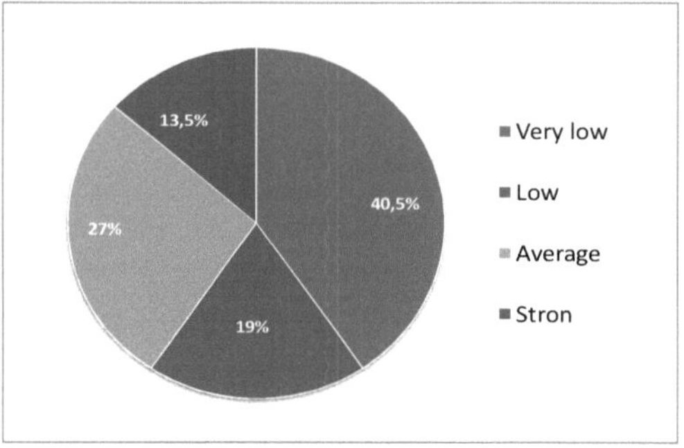

Figure 4: Distribution of participants according to nicotine dependence assessed by the Fagerström test in smokers (N=37)

4. FACTORS ASSOCIATED WITH SMOKING

Bivariate analysis showed that nicotine dependence was inversely correlated with physical demands at work. However, there was a significant positive association between nicotine dependence and frustration at work (Table IV).

Table IV: Bivariate analysis between nicotine dependence using the Fagerström test and perceived workload (n = 37)

Critères du raw NASA-TLX*	Exigence mentale	Exigence physique	Exigence temporelle	Effort	Performance	Frustration
Score de Fagerström	r* = -0,1 p = 0,3	r = -0,5 p = 0,001	r = 0,1 p = 0,5	r=-0,2 p= 0,1	r = -0,1 p = 0,2	r = 0,3 p = 0,03

*raw NASA-TLX: raw National Aeronautics and Space Administration Task Load Index

*r = Pearson correlation coefficient

DISCUSSION

20

Smoking is classed as the leading preventable cause of death in the world. According to the World Health Organisation (WHO), every year it is implicated in the deaths of more than 8 million people and causes preventable illness in tens of millions more [12]. The diseases caused by tobacco are numerous, and no other consumer product is as dangerous [13,14]. Despite all the harmful effects of tobacco, its use is widespread throughout the world. The WHO estimates that the prevalence of smoking is 22.3% of the world's population [15].

In the workplace, smoking is becoming increasingly common. Having an idea of the extent of this scourge and its relationship with work is essential for planning prevention strategies devised by the occupational physician. Our study therefore aims to estimate the prevalence of smoking and the relationship between nicotine dependence and perceived workload among workers in an electricity and gas company in the Sfax region.

1. STRENGTHS AND LIMITATIONS OF THE STUDY

Our research is distinguished by its clear objective: to examine the relationship between perceived workload and smoking. However, one challenge we recognise is the small size of our sample, limiting the generalisability of our results to a wider population. To overcome this limitation, a larger-scale study involving all electricity and gas company workers would be essential. Such an approach would provide more robust and generalisable results, thus offering a a deeper understanding of the relationship between perceived workload and smoking in this specific population. In addition, it is crucial to stress that our study adopts a cross-sectional design, which means that we observe the variables at a single point in time. This methodology allows us to identify associations between perceived workload and smoking, but it does not allow us to establish causal links. In other words, we cannot determine whether perceived workload causes smoking or vice versa. To better understand the temporal dynamics of this relationship, longitudinal studies would be needed, following participants over an extended period to establish causal relationships.Therefore, while acknowledging the merits of our study, we urge caution in interpreting our results, highlighting the need for a more in-depth and longitudinal approach to better understand the relationship between perceived workload and smoking. An expansion of the sample and a longitudinal approach could make a significant contribution to the advancement of knowledge in this field, providing more nuanced information and a more solid basis for guiding public health and workplace interventions.

2. MAIN RESULTS

In our study, the prevalence of smoking was 45.1% in an exclusively male population. This was higher than the WHO estimate for the general population and close to the figure for men. in Tunisia [1,16]. Tunisia is ranked among the top 10 countries with the highest prevalence of male smoking [16,17]. The prevalence of smoking could be influenced by the country's socio-economic level. In fact, smoking prevalence is falling in developed countries and rising sharply in low- and middle-income countries such as the Maghreb [18].

The Fagerström test showed that 40.5% of smokers were moderately to highly dependent on nicotine. Specialised care for these participants should be recommended to ensure that they stop smoking. Nicotine dependence in our study was higher than that of seafarers, where it was low to very low in 89% of cases and high to very high in 10.98% of cases [19]. Our results were consistent with the study by Karakas S. et al. of workers in primary and secondary schools [20]. The differences in nicotine dependence between occupational categories could be explained by the fact that constraints in the workplace could influence workers' nicotine dependence. In our study, we used the raw NASA-TLX questionnaire to assess perceived workload. The overall raw TLX score was 69.2±24.9. This indicates a higher perceived workload than for care staff. In fact, the study which evaluated the perceived workload of neonatal resuscitation among care staff found an overall raw TLX score equal to 34 [21]. This could be explained by the difference between the tasks performed by these two professional categories. On the basis of data in the literature, we attempted to investigate the relationship between smoking and work. Smoking was associated with a high workload in a study of workers at a seaport, an occupational environment where workloads need to be reduced to ensure the effectiveness of tobacco control measures [22].

However, in the bivariate analysis in our study, nicotine dependence was inversely correlated with physical exertion at work. Similarly, Nadell MJ et al. found that only high average weekly physical activity at work was associated with higher smoking rates and that physical activity at work was not associated with the number of cigarettes smoked per day [7]. Furthermore, bivariate analysis showed a significant positive association between nicotine dependence and frustration at work. A similar finding was also reported by Hassani S. et al and Radi et al who found that stress and high mental workload at work were associated with smoking prevalence [23,24]. However, there was no association between work-related stress and nicotine dependence among law enforcement officers in an Indian study [25].

The variation in mood that accompanies physical activity at work has also been suggested as a possible explanation for the link between physical activity at work and smoking [26,27]. In fact, high levels of physical activity at work could be associated with depression, explaining the use of tobacco when physical activity at work is intense [28]. Moderate physical activity at work, on the other hand, was associated with an improvement in mood and hence with the absence of smoking [29,30].

3. RECOMMENDATIONS

In our study, smoking was a prevalent problem. Tobacco control measures are fully justified because they not only prevent a number of diseases but also encourage workers to have a smoke-free workplace. Incorporating awareness-raising into a smoking cessation programme is a proactive and collaborative approach between the occupational physician and the GP. These health professionals play a crucial role in encouraging patients to stop smoking and providing essential support throughout the process. During medical consultations, doctors can incorporate minimal advice on smoking cessation, offering succinct but powerful information on the benefits of stopping smoking and the resources available to help individuals in this process. This minimal advice, although brief, has been shown to be effective in inspiring positive changes in smoking behaviour.A crucial component of this minimal advice is the encouragement to integrate nicotine replacement therapy. Combining minimal advice with nicotine replacement therapy options, such as patches, gum or inhalers, offers a multidimensional approach. for smoking cessation. These therapies help to reduce withdrawal symptoms, thereby improving the chances of a successful cessation process.Involving occupational physicians and GPs in these awareness-raising initiatives strengthens the coordination of care and promotes a holistic approach to smoking cessation. By working together, they can offer ongoing support, adjust strategies according to individual needs and encourage patients to persevere in their journey towards a smoke-free life. This collaboration between healthcare professionals represents a crucial step in the fight against smoking and the promotion of a healthier lifestyle for workers [31].

At national level, a series of initiatives have been deployed to combat smoking, highlighting the commitment to public health. Signing up to the World Health Organisation (WHO) Framework Convention on Tobacco Control is a significant step in this process. This international convention aims to coordinate global efforts to reduce smoking prevalence and protect future generations from the harmful effects of tobacco. Adherence to this convention reflects the country's commitment to adopting public health policies in line with international tobacco control standards. At the same time, national tobacco prevention strategies have been developed to specifically address the challenges associated with tobacco consumption at the national level. These strategies often include awareness-raising campaigns, educational programmes, capacity-building initiatives for health professionals, and regulatory measures to reduce access to and availability of tobacco products. The legal arsenal relating to the ban on smoking in public places is an essential component of this national fight against smoking. These laws aim to protect the health of citizens by creating smoke-free environments in places such as restaurants, bars, workplaces and other public spaces. These regulations help to reduce exposure to passive smoking, promote cessation and create a social culture that discourages smoking. By combining these different actions, the country is demonstrating a comprehensive and integrated approach to preventing and controlling smoking, thereby promoting public health and the quality of life of its citizens. This coordination between adherence to international standards, development of national strategies and implementation of anti-smoking legislation illustrates a sustained commitment to the fight against this major public health problem. [32]. Such actions must be applied with greater rigour and awareness of their effectiveness.

CONCLUSION

Smoking is classed as the leading preventable cause of death in the world. According to the WHO, it is implicated in the deaths of more than 8 million people each year and causes preventable illness in tens of millions more. Smoking continues to emerge in the workplace. Having an idea of the extent of this scourge and its relationship to work is crucial to planning prevention strategies devised by the occupational physician. To this end, we conducted this study among employees of the electricity and gas company in the Sfax region, with the aim of assessing the prevalence of smoking and the relationship between nicotine dependence and perceived workload. We conducted a descriptive and analytical cross-sectional study during the periodic inspection of electrical technicians. The study concerned electrical technicians who agreed to take part in our survey. Incomplete forms were excluded from the survey. Eighty-two male employees participated in our study. The average age was 38.4 ± 10.12 years. Married employees represented 69.5% of the population. The prevalence of smoking was 45.1%. The average number of pack-years (PY) was 13.28±10.72 PY. Seven of the smokers reported using chicha and none used neffa. The average consumption of chicha was 3 ± 3 chichas per week. Nicotine dependence assessed by the Fagerström test was moderate to strong in 40.5% of smokers. The overall raw TLX score was 69.2±24.9. Bivariate analysis showed that nicotine dependence was inversely correlated with physical demands at work. However, there was a significant positive association between nicotine dependence and frustration at work. Smoking among electricity and gas company workers is a prevalent phenomenon. The association of smoking with certain aspects of perceived workload justifies the reinforcement of preventive measures likely to reduce work constraints, in conjunction with anti-smoking actions targeting smoking employees by providing them with comprehensive care.

REFERENCES

1. Alison Commar (WHO Jenewa), Vinayak Prasad (WHO Jenewa) ET d'Espaignet (Universitas N, Australia). WHO global report on trends in prevalence of tobacco use Fourth edition. 2000;26.

2. Kondo T, Nakano Y, Adachi S, Murohara T. Effects of tobacco smoking on cardiovascular disease. Circ J. 2019;83(10):1980-5.

3. Schabath MB, Cote ML. Cancer Progress and Priorities: Lung Cancer. Cancer Epidemiol Biomarkers Prev. 2019 Oct 1;28(10):1563-79.

4. Fakhfakh R, Ben Romdhane H, Hsairi M, Achour N, Nacef T. Trends in tobacco consumption in Tunisia. East Mediterr Heal J. 2000;6(4):678-86.

5. W. Ben Amar, A. Chakroun, M. Zribi, Z. Khemekhem, F. Ben Jemaa SM. Legislative framework for tobacco control in Tunisia: between inadequacies and lack of enforcement. JIM Sfax. 2017;17:21-6.

6. Lin H, Li M, Chen M, Liu Y, Lin Y, Liu Z, et al. The association of workplace smoke-free policies on individual smoking and quitting-related behaviours. BMC Public Health. 2021;21(1):1-7.

7. Nadell MJ, Mermelstein RJ, Hedeker D, Marquez DX. Original investigation Work and Non-Work Physical Activity Predict Real-

Time Smoking Level and Urges in Young Adults. 2015;803-9.

8. Pinsker EA, Hennrikus DJ, Hannan PJ, Lando HA, Brosseau LM. Smoking patterns, quit behaviors, and smoking environment of workers in small manufacturing companies. Am J Ind Med. 2015 Sep 1;58(9):996-1007.

9. Kassim S, Salam M, Croucher R. Validity and reliability of the fagerstrom test for cigarette dependence in a sample of Arabic speaking UK-resident Yemeni khat chewers. Asian Pacific J Cancer Prev. 2012;13(4):1285-8.

10. Ganier F, Hoareau C, Devillers F. Évaluation Des Performances Et De La Charge De Travail Induits Par L'Apprentissage De Procédures De Maintenance En Environnement Virtuel. Trav Hum. 2013;76(4):335-63.

11. Said S, Gozdzik M, Roche TR, Braun J, Rössler J, Kaserer A, et al. Validation of the raw national aeronautics and space administration task load index (NASA-TLX) questionnaire to assess perceived workload in patient monitoring tasks: Pooled analysis study using mixed models. J Med Internet Res. 2020;22(9).

12. WHO report on the global tobacco epidemic, 2021: new and emerging products: executive summary.

13. Tobacco: deadly under all its forms. Available from:

https://apps.who.int/iris/handle/10665/43466

14. Guide to implementing anti-smoking measures. Available from:

https://apps.who.int/iris/handle/10665/43724?locale-

attribute=es&show=full

15. Tobacco.Available from: https://www.who.int/fr/news-room/fact-

sheets/detail/tobacco

16. Edition S. " Tunisian Health Examination. 2019;

17. Health Promotion. Available from:

https://www.who.int/teams/health-promotion/tobacco-control/who-

report-on- the-global-tobacco-epidemic-2019

18. Cigarette Smoking - United States, 2006-2008 and 2009-2010.

Available from:

https://www.cdc.gov/mmwr/preview/mmwrhtml/su6203a14.htm

19. Grappasonni I, Scuri S, Petrelli F, Nguyen CTT, Sibilio F, Canio

M Di, et al. Survey on smoking habits among seafarers. Acta Biomed.

2019;90(4):497-505.

20. Karakas S, Paklarcié M, Kukié E. The Incidence of Smoking

Habits and the Degree of Nicotine Dependence in Education Workers.

Acta Med Acad. 2019 Aug 1;48(2):193-204.

21. Zehnder EC, Law BHY, Schmölzer GM. Assessment of Healthcare Provider Workload in Neonatal Resuscitation. Front Pediatr. 2020 Dec 22; 8:840.

22. Cezar-Vaz MR, Bonow CA, de Almeida MCV, Sant'Anna CF, Cardoso LS. Workload and associated factors: a study in maritime port in Brazil. Rev Lat Am Enfermagem. 2016 ;24.

23. Hassani S, Yazdanparast T, Seyedmehdi SM, Ghaffari M, Attarchi M, Bahadori B. Relationship of occupational and non-occupational stress with smoking in automotive industry workers. Tanaffos. 2014;13(2):35-42.

24. Radi S, Ostry A, LaMontagne AD. Job stress and other working conditions: Relationships with smoking behaviors in a representative sample of working Australians. Am J Ind Med. 2007;50(8):584-96.

25. Priyanka R, Rao A, Rajesh G, Shenoy R, Mithun Pai BH. Work-associated stress and nicotine dependence among law enforcement personnel in Mangalore, India. Asian Pacific J Cancer Prev. 2016;17(2):829-33.

26. Roberts V, Maddison R, Simpson C, Bullen C, Prapavessis H. The acute effects of exercise on cigarette cravings, withdrawal symptoms, affect, and smoking behaviour: Systematic review update and meta-

analysis. Psychopharmacology (Berl). 2012;222(1):1-15.

27. Kaczynski AT, Manske SR, Mannell RC, Grewal K. Smoking and physical activity: a systematic review. Am J Health Behav. 2008 ;32(1):93-110.

28. McKercher CM, Schmidt MD, Sanderson KA, Patton GC, Dwyer T, Venn AJ. Physical Activity and Depression in Young Adults. Am J Prev Med. 2009;36(2):161-4.

29. Poole L, Steptoe A, Wawrzyniak AJ, Bostock S, Mitchell ES, Hamer M. Associations of objectively measured physical activity with daily mood ratings and psychophysiological stress responses in women. Psychophysiology. 2011;48(8):1165-72.

30. Wichers M, Peeters F, Rutten BPF, Jacobs N, Derom C, Thiery E, et al. A time-lagged momentary assessment study on daily life physical activity and affect. Heal Psychol. 2012;31(2):135-44.

31. Rigotti NA, Munafo MR, Stead LF. Smoking cessation interventions for hospitalized smokers: a systematic review. Arch Intern Med. 2008 Oct 10;168(18):1950.

32. Minist T. National Multisectoral Strategy for the Prevention and Control of Noncommunicable Diseases (NCDs). 2018;2018-25.

SUMMARY

Introduction: In the workplace, a smoke-free environment is vital to ensure the health of workers and those around them. Understanding the relationship between smoking and work is a prerequisite for tobacco control measures.

Objective: To assess the prevalence of smoking in an electricity and gas company in the Sfax region (Tunisia) and to study the relationship between workers' nicotine dependence and perceived workload.

Methods: We conducted a cross-sectional descriptive and analytical survey evaluating the smoking behaviour of technical staff at an electricity and gas company. The study was conducted between July and December 2022 using a two-part questionnaire. The first part was completed by the participant and the second by the investigator. Nicotine dependence was assessed by the Fagerström test and perceived workload by the raw NASA-TLX questionnaire.

Results: Our population comprised 82 male technical staff. Active smoking was reported by 45.1% of participants. Nicotine dependence assessed by the Fagerström test was moderate to high in 40.5% of smokers. According to the raw NASA-TLX, the mean values for mental and physical demands were 88.8 ± 13.5 and 63.6 ± 24.7 respectively. Bivariate analysis showed that nicotine dependence was inversely correlated with physical demands at work and positively correlated with frustration at work.

Conclusion: Smoking is common among technical staff at the electricity and gas company. The association between smoking and perceived workload prompts us to take preventive measures relating to working conditions.

Key words: Smoking/ Professional environment / Nicotine dependence / Perceived workload.

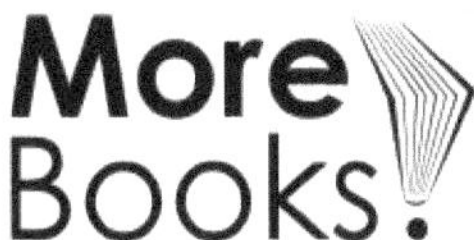

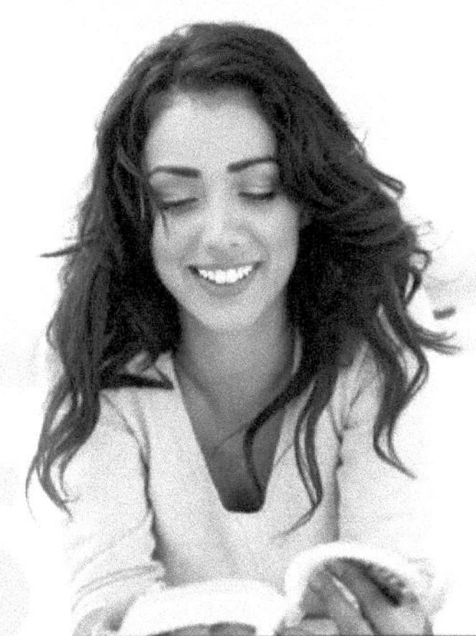

I want morebooks!

Buy your books fast and straightforward online - at one of world's fastest growing online book stores! Environmentally sound due to Print-on-Demand technologies.

Buy your books online at
www.morebooks.shop

Kaufen Sie Ihre Bücher schnell und unkompliziert online – auf einer der am schnellsten wachsenden Buchhandelsplattformen weltweit! Dank Print-On-Demand umwelt- und ressourcenschonend produziert.

Bücher schneller online kaufen
www.morebooks.shop

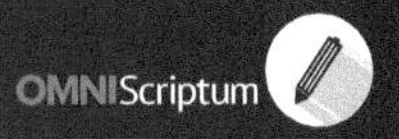

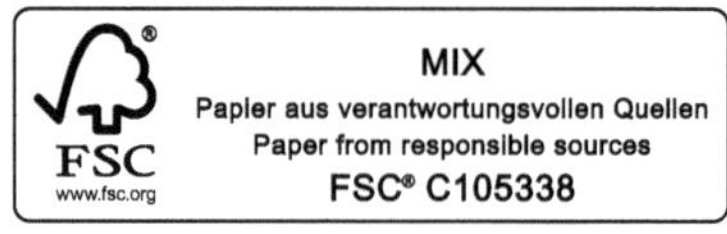

Printed by Books on Demand GmbH, Norderstedt / Germany